Over-50 Women's Bodybuilding Diet

Bodybuilders diet for ladies over 50 and beginners step-by-step

Workout programmes

Dr Lavinia Z. Mark

DISCLAIMER

Copyright © by Dr Lavinia Z. Mark 2023. All rights reserved.

Before this document is duplicated or reproduced in any manner, the publisher's consent must be gained. Therefore, the contents within can neither be stored electronically, transferred, nor kept in a database. Neither in Part nor full can the document be copied, scanned, faxed, or retained without approval from the publisher or creator.

TABLE OF CONTENT

Over-50 Women's Bodybuilding Diet 1
INTRODUCTION 6
CHAPTER 1 7
Understanding the Unique Needs 7
CHAPTER 2 8
Nutrition Fundamentals 8
CHAPTER 3 10
Nutritional Requirements and Changes with Age 10
CHAPTER 4 12
Importance of Macronutrients 12
CHAPTER 5 14
Crafting a Bodybuilding Diet 14
CHAPTER 6 16
Designing a Balanced Meal Plan 16
CHAPTER 7 17
Meal Timing and Frequency 17
CHAPTER 8 19
Adapting Caloric Intake for Muscle Building and Maintenance 19
CHAPTER 9 20
Critical Food Choices and Recipes 20
CHAPTER 10 23
Sample Meal Plans and Recipes 23
CHAPTER 11 25
Hydration and its Impact 25
CHAPTER 12 26
Importance of Hydration for Performance and Recovery 26
CHAPTER 13 28
Hydration Strategies 28

CHAPTER 14..30
Optimizing Training and Nutrition....................................30
CHAPTER 15..31
Synchronizing Diet with Workout Routines 31
CHAPTER 16..32
Pre- and Post-Workout Nutrition Strategies......................32
CHAPTER 17..34
Overcoming Challenges and Adjusting for Hormonal Changes 34
CHAPTER 18..36
Managing Hormonal Changes Effectively Through Diet....................36
CHAPTER 19..38
Techniques for Breaking and Adjusting to Age-Related Difficulties 38
CHAPTER 20..40
Rest and Recovery 40
CONCLUSION 42

In a quiet suburban neighbourhood, **Maria**, a vibrant woman in her 50s, found herself at a crossroads.

Years had passed, and her **passion** for fitness lingered despite life's demands.

She stumbled upon **bodybuilding** tailored for women over 50, a revelation that ignited her spirit anew.

Embarking on this **journey** wasn't just about sculpting muscles; it became a narrative of resilience and newfound empowerment.

With a carefully curated diet as her ally, **Maria** witnessed transformative changes.

Balanced nutrition fortified her body, granting her strength and endurance she hadn't felt in years.

As her muscles grew, so did her confidence and zest for life.

Beyond physical transformation, the diet anchored **Maria** amidst life's tumult.

It wasn't merely about lifting weights but lifting spirits and embracing vitality.

She radiated a contagious energy that inspired her peers through discipline and nourishment, illustrating that age was never a barrier to achieving newfound wellness and inner strength.

INTRODUCTION

Welcome to a revolution in fitness, where age is not a limit but a gateway to redefining strength and vitality.

The Over-50 Women's Bodybuilding Diet is a testament to the power of tailored nutrition, designed to sculpt muscles and reignite the flames of passion and resilience within every woman. This isn't your conventional diet; it's a **roadmap** to rewriting the narrative of ageing. Through this comprehensive guide, discover how nutrition becomes the cornerstone of a transformative journey, empowering women to defy stereotypes and embrace a lifestyle that fosters physical prowess and a profound sense of confidence, energy, and unwavering determination. Join us in uncovering the secret to unlocking a reinvigorated life—one rep, one meal, and one empowered woman at a time.

In a world often fixated on youth, this guide serves as a beacon, illuminating the path for women over 50 to reclaim their strength and rewrite their stories. Beyond mere aesthetics, this isn't about chasing a fleeting idea; it's about embracing a sustainable, holistic approach that celebrates the beauty of maturity and its limitless potential.

Delve into a wealth of nutritional insights, personalized meal plans, and strategies meticulously crafted to cater to the unique needs of women navigating the intricacies of age and fitness. Whether you're a seasoned fitness enthusiast or just stepping into this empowering realm, this guide promises more than physical transformation—it offers a renewed mindset, a rekindled passion, and a community that champions the resilience and grace of every woman on this extraordinary journey.

CHAPTER 1
Understanding the Unique Needs

Understanding the unique needs in bodybuilding is a nuanced exploration that goes beyond the surface of physical training.

It delves into a complex interplay of biological, hormonal, and lifestyle factors defining this pivotal life stage. At this juncture, women often face distinctive challenges—fluctuating hormone levels, changes in metabolism, and the gradual onset of age-related muscle loss. These factors necessitate a tailored approach to nutrition, training, and recovery.

For women over 50, bodybuilding isn't just about building muscle; it's about preserving bone density, enhancing mobility, and cultivating resilience against age-related health concerns.

Their bodies respond differently to exercise and nutrition compared to younger counterparts, necessitating a focus on quality nutrition, adequate protein intake, and strategic training to counteract muscle loss and maintain strength. Moreover, considerations of joint health, recovery optimization, and hormonal fluctuations become paramount.

Embracing this phase with a comprehensive understanding allows for developing targeted training programs and dietary strategies. It's about crafting a holistic approach that doesn't merely aim for aesthetic changes but prioritizes longevity, functional strength, and overall well-being. Recognizing and addressing these unique needs empowers **women over 50** to navigate their bodybuilding journey with precision, grace, and an unwavering commitment to physical and mental vitality.

CHAPTER 2
Nutrition Fundamentals

Nutrition fundamentals in bodybuilding serve as the cornerstone for vitality, strength, and overall well-being. The body undergoes various shifts at this stage, demanding a more tailored approach to dietary intake. Prioritizing macronutrients—proteins, carbohydrates, and fats—takes precedence, but the quality and distribution of these nutrients become pivotal.

Proteins, the building blocks of muscle, are crucial in preserving lean muscle mass. Increasing protein intake helps counteract age-related muscle loss and supports muscle recovery post-exercise.

Concurrently, adequate carbohydrates provide essential energy for workouts and daily activities. Focusing on complex carbohydrates, such as whole grains and vegetables, helps stabilize blood sugar levels and sustain energy throughout the day.

Strategic inclusion of healthy fats, like **omega-3 fatty acids** found in **fish**, **nuts**, and **seeds**, supports joint health, cognitive function, and hormone regulation—particularly pertinent for women over 50. Micronutrients, including calcium, vitamin D, and magnesium, become imperative for bone health and overall vitality.

Moreover, mindful meal timing and portion control are vital. Optimizing nutrient intake throughout the day supports metabolism and aids in muscle recovery. Balancing these fundamentals—adequate protein for muscle preservation, quality carbohydrates for sustained energy, healthy fats for overall health, and micronutrient-rich foods—lays the foundation for a nutrition plan tailored to the unique needs of women over 50 in bodybuilding.

This approach fuels physical performance and fosters resilience, ensuring that each meal is a step towards vitality and strength.

CHAPTER 3

Nutritional Requirements and Changes with Age

As women age, nutritional requirements undergo shifts that necessitate a thoughtful approach to diet and supplementation. Understanding these changes and applying tailored strategies is crucial for optimizing health and fitness in bodybuilding for **women over 50**.

1. Protein Intake: With age, proteins are needed to counteract muscle loss. Aim for higher protein intake spread across meals to support muscle preservation and repair. This typically ranges from 1.2 to 1.7 grams of protein per kilogram of body weight daily, but individual needs may vary.

2. Calcium and Vitamin D: Bone health becomes a priority. Women over 50 need more calcium and vitamin D to maintain bone density. If necessary, incorporate dairy products, leafy greens, fortified foods, and supplements to meet these needs.

3. Fiber-Rich Foods: Digestive health often becomes more sensitive. Prioritize fiber-rich foods such as fruits, vegetables, whole grains, and legumes to aid digestion and promote gut health.

4. Healthy Fats: Hormonal changes may affect lipid metabolism. Opt for healthy fats like avocados, nuts, seeds, and fatty fish to support heart health and hormone regulation.

5. Hydration: Aging can diminish the sensation of thirst, leading to dehydration. Ensure adequate hydration by drinking water consistently throughout the day and consuming hydrating foods like fruits and vegetables.

Applying these changes involves creating a balanced and diverse diet plan that accounts for increased protein intake, focuses on nutrient-dense foods, includes sufficient calcium and vitamin D sources, and emphasizes hydration.

Moreover, consulting with a nutritionist or healthcare provider can help tailor these nutritional adjustments to individual needs and health conditions, ensuring an optimal approach to bodybuilding for women over 50.

CHAPTER 4
Importance of Macronutrients

Macronutrients—proteins, carbohydrates, and fats—play pivotal roles in the body's functionality, especially in optimizing performance in bodybuilding for women over 50.

1. Proteins: Essential for muscle repair and growth, proteins supply amino acids crucial for maintaining lean muscle mass. For women over 50, preserving muscle becomes vital to combat age-related muscle loss.

Protein intake aids in recovery post-exercise and supports overall strength. Sources like lean meats, fish, eggs, dairy, legumes, and plant-based proteins are essential in maintaining adequate protein levels.

2. Carbohydrates: Carbohydrates fuel workouts and daily activities, often regarded as the body's primary energy source. Opt for complex carbohydrates—found in whole grains, fruits, vegetables, and legumes—to sustain energy levels, regulate blood sugar, and support endurance during workouts.

3. Fats: Healthy fats, including omega-3 fatty acids, are crucial for hormone regulation, joint health, and brain function. Incorporate sources like avocados, nuts, seeds, and fatty fish to maintain overall health and support optimal bodily functions.

In addition to macronutrients, micronutrients—such as vitamins and minerals—also play vital roles in performance optimization in bodybuilding for women over 50.

1. Calcium and Vitamin D: Essential for bone health and strength, especially crucial as bone density declines with age. Adequate intake of foods like dairy and leafy greens and exposure to sunlight (for vitamin D synthesis) are vital.

2. Magnesium and Potassium: Important for muscle function and recovery. Foods like bananas, spinach, nuts, and seeds are excellent sources.

Supplements can be beneficial for filling nutritional gaps, especially in cases where dietary intake might be insufficient. For **women over 50 in bodybuilding**, supplements like **protein powders, vitamin D, calcium, omega-3 fatty acids**, and multivitamins tailored to their specific needs can complement a balanced diet and aid in optimal performance and overall health.

However, consulting with a healthcare professional or nutritionist before incorporating supplements is crucial to ensure they align with individual health requirements.

CHAPTER 5
Crafting a Bodybuilding Diet

Crafting a bodybuilding diet involves a strategic approach tailored to their unique needs and goals.

Here's an essential process to create such a diet plan:

1. Assessment of Individual Needs: Begin by assessing individual health status, fitness goals, activity levels, and any specific dietary restrictions or health concerns. Consulting with a nutritionist or healthcare professional can provide valuable insights into personalized requirements.

2. Determining Caloric Needs: Calculate daily caloric needs based on factors such as basal metabolic rate (BMR), activity level, and goals—whether it's maintaining, gaining, or losing weight. Online calculators or professional guidance can aid in this calculation.

3. Protein Prioritization: Given the importance of protein in preserving muscle mass, ensure sufficient protein intake. Set a target based on individual factors, aiming for a range between 1.2 to 1.7 grams per kilogram of body weight.

4. Balancing Macronutrients: Distribute macronutrients—proteins, carbohydrates, and fats—strategically throughout the day. Emphasize lean proteins, complex carbohydrates, and healthy fats in meals to support energy levels, muscle preservation, and overall health.

5. Meal Planning and Timing: Structure meals to align with training schedules, emphasizing pre-and post-workout nutrition. Prioritize whole, nutrient-dense foods and consider smaller, frequent meals to maintain energy levels and aid digestion.

6. Hydration Strategy: Incorporate ample water intake throughout the day. Hydration is crucial for performance, recovery, and overall health, mainly as ageing may reduce the sensation of thirst.

7. Micronutrient-rich foods: Ensure the diet includes a variety of fruits, vegetables, whole grains, and sources rich in essential vitamins and minerals, catering to bone health, immunity, and overall vitality.

8. Supplementation, if Necessary: Consider supplements to fill potential nutrient gaps. Supplements like protein powders, omega-3 fatty acids, vitamin D, or multivitamins can complement the diet but should be used judiciously and with professional guidance.

9. Monitoring and Adjusting: Regularly assess progress, energy levels, and how the body responds to the diet. Adjustments may be necessary based on individual responses, goals, and any changes in health or activity levels.

Remember, consistency and flexibility are key. Crafting a bodybuilding diet for women over 50 requires a personalized, adaptable approach supporting fitness goals and overall health, ensuring sustainable progress and vitality. Consulting with a healthcare professional or registered dietitian can provide tailored guidance and support.

CHAPTER 6
Designing a Balanced Meal Plan

Designing a balanced meal plan in bodybuilding involves a holistic approach that caters to individual needs, supports muscle preservation, and fosters overall health and vitality.

The process begins with a comprehensive assessment of personal goals, dietary preferences, and nutritional requirements. Start by determining caloric needs based on activity levels and desired outcomes—maintaining weight, building muscle, or losing fat.

Prioritize lean proteins like chicken, fish, tofu, or legumes to support muscle maintenance and repair. Distribute carbohydrates from whole grains, fruits, and vegetables across meals to sustain energy levels, and incorporate healthy fats from sources like avocados, nuts, and olive oil to aid in hormone regulation and overall health.

Strive for variety and balance, incorporating micronutrient-rich foods such as leafy greens, colourful vegetables, and fruits to ensure an adequate intake of vitamins and minerals.

Plan meals strategically around workouts, focusing on pre- and post-exercise nutrition to optimize performance and recovery.

Regularly assess and adjust the meal plan based on individual responses, ensuring it aligns with fitness and long-term health objectives.

Consulting with a nutritionist or registered dietitian can provide invaluable guidance in tailoring a meal plan that suits individual needs and promotes sustained success in bodybuilding for **women over 50**.

CHAPTER 7
Meal Timing and Frequency

Meal timing and frequency are pivotal components in the bodybuilding journey for women over 50, significantly influencing performance, recovery, and overall well-being. The strategic timing of meals orchestrates a symphony within the body, optimizing energy levels and supporting muscle maintenance.

Balancing nutrient intake throughout the day, focusing on regular, smaller meals, helps sustain metabolism and stabilizes blood sugar levels, which is crucial for sustained energy and avoiding energy dips.

Moreover, meal timing around workouts—prioritizing pre- and post-exercise nutrition—becomes instrumental in maximizing performance and facilitating efficient recovery.

This approach ensures the body receives the essential nutrients needed to fuel workouts and initiate muscle repair post-exercise.

Additionally, adequate meal frequency throughout the day prevents overeating or undereating, promotes better digestion, and helps in nutrient absorption.

Understanding the significance of meal timing and frequency enables women over 50 to cultivate a sustainable eating pattern that supports their bodybuilding goals and fosters lasting vitality and overall health.

By strategically spacing meals and snacks, women over 50 can maintain a steady stream of nutrients, aiding in sustained energy levels and supporting their body's demands during workouts and daily activities.

Each meal or snack becomes an opportunity to nourish the body, fortifying it with the essential building blocks for strength and recovery. Moreover, this approach helps regulate appetite and prevents extreme hunger, leading to more mindful eating habits.

Consistency in meal timing establishes a rhythm that optimizes metabolism, aids nutrient utilization, and supports the body's natural processes.

For women venturing into bodybuilding, understanding the importance of meal timing and frequency not only shapes their physical performance but also becomes a cornerstone for nurturing a balanced, sustainable lifestyle that embraces strength, vitality, and holistic well-being at every stage of their journey.

CHAPTER 8

Adapting Caloric Intake for Muscle Building and Maintenance

Adapting caloric intake for muscle building and maintenance among women over 50 in bodybuilding involves a delicate balance between fueling workouts and supporting the body's unique needs for sustained vitality.

Calculating an appropriate caloric surplus or deficit based on individual goals—muscle gain or maintenance—becomes pivotal.

For muscle building, a slight caloric surplus, typically ranging from 250 to 500 extra calories per day, can provide the energy needed to support intense workouts and facilitate muscle growth.

This surplus should be accompanied by a higher intake of quality proteins, ensuring the body has adequate building blocks for muscle repair and growth.

Conversely, when aiming for maintenance or fat loss, a slight deficit in calories—around 250 to 500 fewer calories per day—can encourage gradual fat loss while preserving lean muscle mass.

Adjusting caloric intake is a dynamic process that requires monitoring progress, listening to the body's cues, and making gradual adjustments to ensure a sustainable approach that nurtures muscle growth and overall health for women over 50 in their bodybuilding endeavours.

CHAPTER 9

Critical Food Choices and Recipes

Here are some critical food choices and simple recipes tailored in bodybuilding, focusing on nutrient-dense meals that support muscle maintenance and overall health:

Protein Sources:

Grilled Lemon Herb Chicken:

• Mix a zesty marinade with lemon juice, olive oil, garlic, and your favourite herbs.

• Give your chicken breasts a good soak in this flavorful mix for a few hours.

• Fire up the grill and cook those marinated breasts until they're juicy and charred.

• Serve with steamed veggies and a scoop of quinoa for a deliciously satisfying meal!

Baked Salmon with Avocado Salsa:

• Season your salmon fillets with herbs, a salt pinch, and a pepper sprinkle.

• Pop them into the oven and bake until tender and flaky.

• Meanwhile, prepare a fresh salsa using diced avocado, tomatoes, onions, cilantro, lime juice, and olive oil.

• Once your salmon is done, top it with this vibrant avocado salsa for a burst of flavour to make your taste buds dance!

Essential Carbohydrates:

Quinoa Salad with Chickpeas and Vegetables:

- Cook up a batch of quinoa and toss it with some cooked chickpeas, diced cucumbers, bell peppers, cherry tomatoes, and freshly chopped parsley.

- Drizzle on a light vinaigrette made with olive oil, lemon juice, and a hint of honey.

- It's a vibrant and tasty salad packed with nutrients and textures!

Sweet Potato and Black Bean Tacos:

- Roast those sweet potato cubes with olive oil and your favourite spices until golden and tender.

- Fill up your soft tacos with roasted sweet potatoes, black beans, shredded lettuce, diced onions, and a dollop of Greek yoghurt.

- Get ready to wrap your taste buds around these flavorful and satisfying tacos!

Healthy Fats:

Avocado and Spinach Smoothie Bowl:

- Blend together a creamy mix of avocado, spinach, banana, Greek yoghurt, and almond milk until it's nice and smooth.

- Pour it into a bowl and get creative with the toppings—add some sliced fruits, nuts, seeds, and a drizzle of honey for a delightful breakfast treat!

Almond-Crusted Baked Chicken:

- Coat your chicken breasts with an almond meal, your favourite herbs, and olive oil.

- Bake them until they're beautifully golden and crispy.

- Serve these deliciously nutty chicken breasts with roasted vegetables for a wholesome and satisfying dinner!

These recipes offer versatile and flavorful bodybuilding options for women over 50, providing a balance of macronutrients to fuel workouts, aid recovery, and promote overall health.

Adjust portion sizes and ingredients according to individual nutritional needs and preferences.

CHAPTER 10
Sample Meal Plans and Recipes

Here's a sample meal plan tailored for women over 50 in bodybuilding, accompanied by recipes and preparation instructions:

Day 1:

Breakfast:

- **Avocado and Spinach Smoothie Bowl:**

• Blend together 1 ripe avocado, a handful of spinach, one banana, 1/2 cup Greek yoghurt, and a splash of almond milk until it's smooth and creamy.

• Pour it into a bowl and top it off with sliced strawberries, almonds, and a drizzle of honey for that extra sweetness.

Lunch:

- **Quinoa Salad with Chickpeas and Veggies:**

• Cook up a batch of quinoa and toss it with some cooked chickpeas, diced cucumbers, colourful bell peppers, cherry tomatoes, and chopped parsley.

• Give it a slight drizzle of a simple vinaigrette made of olive oil, lemon juice, and a hint of honey to bring out those flavours.

Dinner:

- **Grilled Lemon Herb Chicken:**

• Get those chicken breasts swimming in a zesty mix of lemon juice, olive oil, garlic, and your favourite herbs.

- Throw them on the grill until they're perfectly cooked, and serve them with steamed broccoli and a side of quinoa. That's a wholesome dinner right there!

Day 2:

Breakfast:

• Greek Yogurt Parfait:

- Take some Greek yoghurt and layer it with a mix of your favourite berries, crunchy granola, and a sprinkle of those healthy chia seeds. It's a tasty, protein-packed start to your day!

Lunch:

• Sweet Potato and Black Bean Tacos:

- Roast sweet potato cubes with olive oil and your favourite spices until golden and delicious.

- Stuff them into soft tacos with black beans, shredded lettuce, diced onions, and a dollop of Greek yoghurt. Tacos are always a hit!

Dinner:

• Baked Salmon with Avocado Salsa:

- Season your salmon fillets with herbs, a pinch of salt, and a sprinkle of pepper, then bake them up until they're perfectly flaky.

- Meanwhile, whip up a vibrant salsa with diced avocado, tomatoes, onions, cilantro, lime juice, and olive oil. Pour it over the salmon for a burst of fresh flavour!

These meal ideas are meant to be simple, tasty, and packed with the good stuff to keep you feeling great and energized throughout your bodybuilding journey! Adjust them to suit your tastes, and enjoy every bite!

CHAPTER 11
Hydration and its Impact

Hydration is an unsung hero in bodybuilding for women over 50, wielding a profound impact beyond mere thirst-quenching. Adequate hydration isn't just about drinking water; it's about sustaining the body's intricate functions, optimizing performance, and aiding recovery.

For women in bodybuilding, proper hydration ensures optimal muscle function, joint lubrication, and temperature regulation during workouts, enhancing endurance and preventing fatigue.

Moreover, it aids in nutrient transport, ensuring vital elements efficiently reach muscles for repair and growth.

Beyond the gym, staying hydrated supports metabolic processes aids digestion, and promotes more apparent cognition—crucial aspects often overlooked in the pursuit of fitness.

For women over 50, where the sensation of thirst might diminish with age, conscientious attention to hydration becomes paramount, as it maintains overall vitality, fosters skin elasticity, and supports joint health.

Embracing hydration as a cornerstone of their regimen empowers women in bodybuilding to elevate their performance, nurture their bodies, and fortify their overall well-being, exemplifying that a simple yet often underestimated act holds the key to enhanced endurance, recovery, and vitality.

CHAPTER 12

Importance of Hydration for Performance and Recovery

Here are key points outlining the significance of hydration for both performance during workouts and the recovery process:

Importance of Hydration for Performance:

1. Maintains Fluid Balance: Adequate hydration ensures the body maintains fluid balance, optimizing cellular function and supporting muscle contraction during workouts. It helps prevent dehydration, which can lead to reduced endurance and performance.

2. Regulates Body Temperature: Proper hydration assists in regulating body temperature, especially during intense physical activities. It helps dissipate heat through sweating, preventing overheating and maintaining optimal performance levels.

3. Sustains Energy Levels: Hydration is crucial in nutrient and oxygen transport to muscles, supporting energy production during workouts. Well-hydrated muscles are more efficient and can perform better, enhancing overall endurance.

Importance of Hydration for Recovery:

1. Facilitates Nutrient Delivery: Adequate hydration post-exercise aids in efficiently transporting nutrients to muscle tissues, enabling quicker recovery.

It replenishes glycogen stores and delivers essential nutrients for muscle repair and growth.

2. Reduces Muscle Soreness: Proper hydration helps flush out metabolic waste products and toxins accumulated during exercise, reducing the likelihood and severity of muscle soreness and stiffness.

3. Supports Tissue Repair: Hydration is essential for optimal cellular function and the repair of damaged tissues. It promotes the healing process, aiding in the repair of micro-tears in muscle fibres caused by exercise.

4. Enhances Recovery Time: Rehydrating adequately after workouts speeds up recovery, allowing the body to recover more efficiently and be ready for subsequent training sessions.

Ensuring consistent **hydration** by drinking water regularly throughout the day, monitoring urine colour to gauge hydration levels, and considering electrolyte intake during intense workouts are vital strategies to support performance and optimize recovery in bodybuilding for women over 50.

CHAPTER 13
Hydration Strategies

Hydration strategies are crucial to support performance, recovery, and overall health.

Here are effective strategies and explanations for optimal hydration:

1. Consistent Water Intake:

Encouraging regular water intake throughout the day is essential. As individuals age, the sensation of thirst might diminish, making it easy to overlook hydration needs. Drinking water consistently helps maintain fluid balance, supports cellular function, and regulates temperature during workouts.

2. Monitoring Urine Color:

One effective method to assess hydration status is by monitoring urine colour. A light yellow or pale colour generally indicates adequate hydration, while darker shades suggest dehydration. Encouraging women over 50 to monitor their urine colour can be a simple yet effective way to gauge their hydration levels.

3. Electrolyte Balance:

Maintaining a balance of electrolytes, such as sodium, potassium, and magnesium, is crucial, especially during intense workouts. Electrolytes aid in fluid absorption and retention, preventing dehydration. Including electrolyte-rich foods or drinks, like coconut water or electrolyte-enhanced beverages, can support hydration and electrolyte balance.

4. Pre- and Post-Workout Hydration:

Encouraging adequate hydration before, during, and after workouts is critical. Pre-workout hydration primes the body for exercise while maintaining hydration during exercise supports performance. Post-workout hydration is vital for replenishing fluids lost through sweating and aiding recovery.

5. Hydrating Foods:

Encouraging the consumption of hydrating foods can also contribute to overall hydration levels. Fruits and vegetables with high water content, such as watermelon, cucumber, oranges, and celery, provide hydration, essential nutrients and antioxidants.

6. Individualized Hydration Plans:

Recognizing that hydration needs vary among individuals, it's crucial to emphasize personalized hydration plans. Factors like body weight, activity level, environmental conditions, and individual sweat rates should be considered when devising a hydration strategy tailored to each woman's unique needs.

These strategies promote consistent and adequate fluid intake, maintain electrolyte balance, and align hydration with workout routines to optimize performance, support recovery, and safeguard overall health.

By adopting these strategies, women can proactively manage their hydration needs, ensuring they stay adequately hydrated throughout their bodybuilding journey.

CHAPTER 14
Optimizing Training and Nutrition

Optimizing training and nutrition stands as the cornerstone, intertwining these elements to achieve peak performance, sustain muscle strength, and foster overall well-being.

Tailoring training regimens to suit individual capabilities and goals is pivotal, focusing on progressive resistance training to preserve and build muscle while accommodating age-related considerations.

Concurrently, nutrition is crucial, emphasizing adequate protein intake for muscle repair and growth, complex carbohydrates for sustained energy, and healthy fats for overall health.

Aligning training schedules with nutrient timing ensures the body receives the necessary fuel before and after workouts, optimizing performance and facilitating effective recovery.

By harmonizing these aspects, women over 50 can harness the synergy between training and nutrition, creating a holistic approach that enhances physical prowess and fortifies their resilience, vitality, and capacity to thrive in bodybuilding.

CHAPTER 15

Synchronizing Diet with Workout Routines

Synchronizing diet with workout routines is a strategic dance, a choreography that optimizes performance, supports recovery, and fuels progress in bodybuilding for women over 50.

It's about crafting a nutritional symphony that harmonizes with the demands of different workouts.

Pre-workout nutrition becomes a cue, offering a balance of carbohydrates and protein for sustained energy and muscle support.

Post-workout nourishment takes the spotlight, providing a mix of protein and carbohydrates to aid muscle repair and replenish glycogen stores.

Throughout the day, meals and snacks maintain the rhythm, ensuring a steady stream of nutrients to support metabolism and recovery.

This synchronization is an art, allowing to elevate their workouts and fuel their bodies in a way that enhances performance and nurtures strength, endurance, and overall vitality.

CHAPTER 16
Pre- and Post-Workout Nutrition Strategies

Pre- and post-workout nutrition are vital strategies, optimizing performance and aiding recovery.

Pre-Workout Nutrition Strategies:

1. Balanced Meal Timing: Consume a balanced meal containing carbohydrates and protein about 1-2 hours before a workout. This meal provides energy and amino acids for muscle support during exercise.

2. Carbohydrates for Energy: Emphasize complex carbohydrates, such as whole grains, fruits, or starchy vegetables, to fuel workouts. They provide a steady release of energy to sustain performance.

3. Protein for Muscle Support: Include a moderate amount of protein, like lean meats, Greek yoghurt, or plant-based sources, to support muscle maintenance and repair during exercise.

4. Hydration: Ensure adequate hydration by drinking water before workouts to prevent dehydration and maintain optimal performance.

Post-Workout Nutrition Strategies:

1. Protein and Carbohydrates Combo: Consume a meal or snack within 30 minutes to an hour post-exercise. This meal should include protein and carbohydrates to replenish glycogen stores and initiate muscle recovery.

2. Lean Protein Sources: Opt for easily digestible protein sources like whey protein, eggs, or chicken to kickstart muscle repair.

3. Carbohydrates for Recovery: Pair protein with carbohydrates to replenish muscle glycogen and enhance recovery. This combination supports efficient nutrient delivery to muscles.

4. Hydration and Electrolytes: Rehydrate with water and consider beverages containing electrolytes to replace fluids lost during exercise and aid recovery.

Strategically planning pre-and post-workout nutrition for women over 50 in bodybuilding supports energy levels during workouts, facilitates muscle repair, and ensures the body has the necessary nutrients to optimize recovery.

CHAPTER 17

Overcoming Challenges and Adjusting for Hormonal Changes

Navigating hormonal changes presents a unique set of challenges that require a thoughtful approach and adaptability.

Hormonal fluctuations, especially during menopause, can impact energy levels, muscle mass, and recovery, affecting their bodybuilding journey.

Overcoming these challenges involves several strategies:

1. Training Adjustments:

- **Tailored Workouts:** Modify training routines to accommodate fluctuations in energy levels. Some days may require lower intensity workouts or more rest days to adapt to hormonal shifts.

- **Focus on Strength Training:** Prioritize resistance training to counteract age-related muscle loss and maintain strength. Incorporate exercises that target bone density, such as weight-bearing exercises.

2. Nutrition Modifications:

- **Protein Intake:** Ensure sufficient protein intake for muscle repair and maintenance. Adjust protein consumption based on individual needs and goals.

- **Balanced Diet:** Emphasize nutrient-dense foods, including sources rich in calcium, vitamin D, and omega-3 fatty acids, to support bone health and overall well-being.

3. Recovery and Rest:

- **Quality Sleep:** Prioritize adequate sleep as it aids in hormone regulation and supports recovery. Aim for consistent and quality sleep to optimize overall health.

- **Stress Management:** Incorporate stress-reducing activities such as yoga, meditation, or relaxation techniques to manage stress, which can impact hormonal balance.

4. Consultation and Adaptability:

- **Healthcare Guidance:** Consult healthcare professionals or specialists to address specific hormonal concerns and tailor strategies accordingly.

- **Flexibility and Adaptation:** Remain flexible and adaptive in training and nutrition plans, adjusting as needed to accommodate hormonal changes and individual responses.

5. Mindset and Persistence:

- **Positive Mindset:** Maintain a positive attitude and be patient with the body's changes. Understand that progress might require more time and adaptation.

- **Consistency:** Stay consistent with workouts and nutrition plans, even during challenging periods. Consistency fosters long-term success and resilience.

By adopting a holistic approach that integrates tailored workouts, balanced nutrition, adequate rest, and adaptability to hormonal changes, you can overcome challenges and continue thriving in their bodybuilding journey, supporting physical and emotional well-being.

Consulting with healthcare professionals and embracing a patient, persistent mindset remains pivotal in navigating these changes effectively.

CHAPTER 18

Managing Hormonal Changes Effectively Through Diet

Here's how dietary choices can help:

1. Balanced Macronutrients:

• **Protein Richness:** Ensure adequate protein intake for muscle maintenance and repair. Lean meats, fish, eggs, dairy, legumes, and plant-based protein sources are beneficial.

• **Healthy Fats:** Incorporate sources of healthy fats like avocados, nuts, seeds, and olive oil, which aid in hormone production and support overall health.

• **Complex Carbohydrates:** Opt for whole grains, fruits, and vegetables as primary carbohydrate sources, providing sustained energy and aiding mood regulation.

2. Phytoestrogenic Foods:

• **Soy-based Products:** Incorporate moderate amounts of soy products like tofu, tempeh, or edamame, which contain phytoestrogens that may help alleviate some menopausal symptoms.

3. Omega-3 Fatty Acids:

• **Fatty Fish and Seeds:** Consume sources rich in omega-3 fatty acids, such as salmon, mackerel, flaxseeds, and chia seeds, known to support hormonal balance and reduce inflammation.

4. Calcium and Vitamin D:

- **Dairy or Alternatives:** Ensure adequate calcium intake from dairy or fortified plant-based alternatives to support bone health.

- **Sun Exposure and Supplements:** Get enough vitamin D through safe sun exposure or supplements, as it aids in calcium absorption and supports hormonal function.

5. Limiting Caffeine and Alcohol:

- **Moderation:** Reduce consumption of caffeine and alcohol, which can exacerbate hormonal fluctuations and disrupt sleep patterns.

6. Hydration and Antioxidants:

- **Water Intake:** Maintain proper hydration levels to support overall bodily functions and hormone regulation.

- **Antioxidant-rich Foods:** Include fruits, vegetables, and green tea, which contain antioxidants that may help reduce oxidative stress associated with hormonal changes.

7. Consulting a Nutritionist:

- **Individualized Approach:** Consider consulting a nutritionist or healthcare professional to create a personalized diet plan that addresses specific hormonal concerns and individual needs.

8. Stress Management:

- **Mindfulness and Relaxation:** Incorporate stress-reducing practices like meditation, yoga, or deep breathing exercises to manage stress, which can impact hormonal balance.

By focusing on a nutrient-dense, balanced diet that includes essential macronutrients, phytoestrogenic foods, omega-3 fatty acids, adequate calcium and vitamin D while minimizing caffeine and alcohol intake.

CHAPTER 19

Techniques for Breaking and Adjusting to Age-Related Difficulties

With these bodybuilding tactics, you can efficiently manage age-related obstacles and plateaus:

1. Gradual Overload and Diverse Exercise Programs:

• Modify Workout Routine: To avoid plateaus, vary the workouts, levels of intensity, and training techniques. By progressively raising the weights or resistance, incorporate progressive overload.

• Emphasize functional movements that improve balance, flexibility, and joint stability while enhancing daily tasks. This is known as functional training.

2. Rest and Recuperation:

• Put Recovery First: Give yourself enough time off between sessions to promote muscle growth and regeneration. Think about combining low-impact exercises like yoga or swimming with active recuperation days.

• Quality Sleep: Get enough sleep; it's essential for healing and hormone balance. Strive for regular, peaceful sleep schedules.

3. Hydration and Nutrition:

- Nutrient-Dense Diet: To promote muscle growth and general health, keep a well-balanced diet high in protein, good fats, and complex carbohydrates.

- Hydration: Drink enough water throughout the day to aid digestion, healing, and cellular function.

4. Adaptability and Mentality:

- Mind-Muscle Connection: Pay attention to your body's mental and physical connections to ensure your targeted muscle groups' correct form and activation.

- Optimistic mindset: Have an optimistic outlook while acknowledging that age-related variables may cause progress to take longer. Remain tenacious and acknowledge little accomplishments.

5. Observation and Modification:

- Regular Assessment: Keep tabs on development, assess performance, and modify diet and exercise regimens in response to individual needs.

- Consult Experts: To create customized programs that take age-related changes into account, get advice from nutritionists, physical therapists, or fitness coaches.

6. Perseverance and Patience:

- Consistency: Even when results appear sluggish, continue with your exercise and diet regimens. Consistency leads to improvements over time.

- Patience and Adaptation: Accept the trip, realizing that it could take some time and flexibility to adjust to changes brought on by ageing.

Women over 50 can effectively overcome age-related obstacles and plateaus by incorporating various workouts, prioritizing recovery, maintaining a balanced diet, cultivating a positive mindset, and seeking help when necessary. These strategies will ensure that their bodybuilding adventure continues.

CHAPTER 20

Rest and Recovery

Rest and recovery are indispensable components of a successful bodybuilding regimen and here's why they're crucial and how to optimize them.

Importance of Rest:

1. Muscle Repair: Rest allows muscles to recover and repair after strenuous workouts, aiding muscle growth and adaptation.

2. Hormonal Balance: Quality rest contributes to hormonal balance, supporting muscle recovery and overall well-being.

3. Injury Prevention: Ample rest reduces the risk of overuse injuries, providing time for the body to heal and preventing burnout.

Strategies for Optimal Rest and Recovery:

1. Adequate Sleep: Aim for 7-9 hours of sleep per night to facilitate muscle repair, hormone regulation, and overall recovery.

2. Active Recovery: Incorporate light activities like walking, yoga, or swimming on rest days to enhance blood flow and aid muscle recovery without taxing the body.

3. Hydration: Maintain proper hydration levels to support bodily functions and recovery processes.

4. Nutrient-Dense Diet: Consume a balanced diet rich in proteins, healthy fats, and carbohydrates to provide the necessary nutrients for recovery.

5. Stress Management: Employ stress-reduction techniques like meditation, deep breathing exercises, or hobbies to manage stress levels, supporting recovery.

6. Periodization: Incorporate planned periods of deloading or reduced training intensity to allow for extended recovery and prevent overtraining.

Listening to Your Body:

Understanding and responding to individual signals from the body is crucial. Experiencing excessive fatigue, persistent soreness, or decreased performance might indicate the need for additional rest or adjustments in training intensity.

Balancing Training and Rest:

Finding the optimal balance between training and rest is vital. While workouts stimulate muscle growth, rest is where the body repairs and strengthens. Incorporating adequate rest periods into a training program is essential for long-term progress and overall health.

Rest and recovery are not merely breaks from training; they are integral parts of the bodybuilding process, facilitating muscle repair, growth, and overall well-being.

CONCLUSION

The journey transcends mere physical fitness, embodying a holistic pursuit of strength, resilience, and well-being.

Balancing bodybuilding aspirations with overall health necessitates a harmonious fusion of mindful training, nourishing nutrition, adequate rest, and a profound respect for the body's evolving needs.

It's about setting realistic goals that honour individual capabilities, fostering a mindset that values progress and well-being, and embracing a diversified approach to fitness that encompasses physical strength, mental fortitude, and emotional balance.

This journey isn't solely about sculpting muscles; it's about nurturing a lifestyle that exudes vitality, celebrates every achievement, and gracefully adapts to age-related changes.

By embracing this holistic ethos, women over 50 embarking on the bodybuilding path can find empowerment, resilience, and a profound sense of well-being that transcends the confines of the gym, enriching their lives in multifaceted ways.

Printed in the USA
CPSIA information can be obtained
at www.ICGtesting.com
LVHW012200281223
767704LV00050B/2120